KETO DIET INSTANT POT

POT

Cookbook

ISBN-13: 978-1729730263
ISBN-10: 1729730264

Interior, Front and Back Cover Design by Amy Walker

Printed in the United States of America.

First Edition

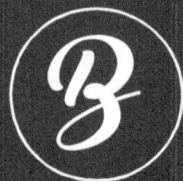

Jolly Books Hub

CONTENTS

Breakfast Recipes

Lunch Recipes

Chicken, Pork, Lamb and Beef Recipes

Side Dishes, Snacks, and Appetizer Recipes

Dessert Recipes

Cooking Notes

AUTHOR

"To my dearest Daniel"

A graduate of UCLA, Amy Walker M.D. earned her bachelor's degree in Health and Nutrition in 1992. She is a passionate advocate for the ketogenic diet and the health benefits it offers to millions of people worldwide. After a highly successful career helping millions of people lose weight, Amy has now retired gracefully to Los Angeles, CA. Every month Amy likes to give back to society by hosting ketogenic diet classes to help people lose weight in her local community. In her free time, Amy likes cooking, blogging, walking her two dogs Toby and Arthur and spending time with friends and family.

... Amy

Ketogenic 101

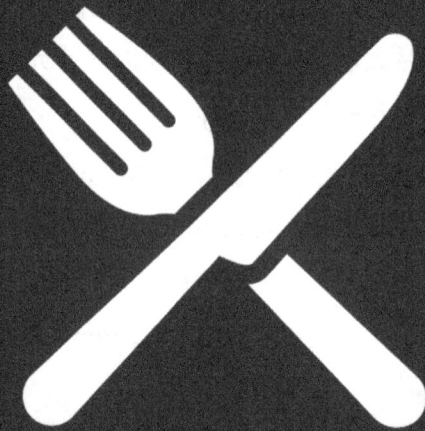

Keto 101

What is the Ketogenic Diet?

Unlike many other diets, this one is easy to understand! The ketogenic diet is simply a high fat, low carbohydrate diet that involves reducing your intake of carbs and replacing them with fats. When you eat foods that are high in carbs, your body produces two things: insulin and glucose.

✓ **Glucose** is a molecule needed by our bodies to convert and use the energy from the food we eat to fuel our body, typically carbohydrate.

✓ **Insulin** is a substance made by our pancreas to process glucose within our bloodstream.

Since glucose is our main source of energy, the fat we have stored away is therefore not needed and sits there unused. When deciding if the ketogenic diet is for them, many people choose a typical diet of eating foods high in carbs. We have been taught that carbs are needed for energy since we were tots. This is true, but only to a point.

Despite what you may have read, there are four types of ketogenic diet.

✓ High-Protein Ketogenic Diet: This type of keto diet involves eating lots of protein. The ratio required to stick to this type of diet is 60% fat, 35% protein and 5% carbohydrates.

- ✓ Targeted Ketogenic Diet (Tkd): If you like the freedom of having some room to move around on a diet, this one is for you! You can intake more carbs if you are working out as well.
- ✓ Cyclical Ketogenic Diet (Ckd): This type requires periods of high-carb intake—for example, 5 ketogenic days paired with a few high-carb consumption days.
- ✓ Standard Ketogenic Diet (Skd): This type of keto diet is the most popular and recommended. It requires you to consume moderate amounts of protein and high amounts of fat. It is based around this popular macro: 75% fat, 20% protein and 5% carbs.

The standard ketogenic diet is the most popular diet for beginners, but you may find that the other three diets are better suited to your body and personal goals. For now, however, I suggest that you start with the standard ketogenic diet to see how your body adapts and to minimize any side affects you may experience on the diet. Many of my students also start with the standard diet and their weight loss results have been excellent because they have exceeded my expectations every time.

History of the Ketogenic Diet

The ketogenic diet has a long and rich history, predating most of the diet trends and fads on the market today. Beginning in the 1920s and 1930s, an early form of the ketogenic diet was used to treat patients with epilepsy. This was the only help patients had until medications were developed in later years—for example, insulin injections. An interesting fact is that in 20% to 30% of all cases, the ketogenic diet remains more effective than medications in treating epilepsy. Today, despite our medical advancements, the ketogenic diet is still used by practitioners as an alternative remedy for treating epilepsy.

In slightly more technical terms, in 1921, an endocrinologist by the name of Rollin Woodyatt, discovered that the ketogenic diet enables our liver to produce three water-soluble compounds. These are:

- ✓ β-hydroxybutyrate
- ✓ acetoacetate
- ✓ acetone

Together, these compounds are known as ketone bodies. During the early 20th Century, an American by the name of Bernarr Macfadden introduced fasting as a means of improving health and wellbeing. His student osteopath, Hugh Conklin, then introduced fasting as a treatment to control epilepsy. Coklin proposed that epileptic seizures are caused by a toxin secreted in the intestine and suggested that fasting for 18 to 25 days could cause the toxin to disappear completely. His epileptic patients were put on a 'water diet', which he reported cured both children and adults with the condition. An analysis of the study performed showed that 20% of Coklin's patients became seizure-free, while 50% demonstrated remarkable improvement. Fasting therapy was soon adopted as part of mainstream therapy for epilepsy and in 1916, Dr McMurray reported to the New York Medical Journal that he had successfully treated epileptic patients by prescribing fasting, followed by a diet free of starch and sugar.

Moving on to the 1960s, Russel Wilder, a medical student, coined the phrase 'ketogenic diet' for its official use in the treatment of epilepsy. After considerable research in the 1960s, scientists found that medium-chain triglycerides produced even more ketones per unit of energy. This led to a revised ketogenic diet for epilepsy patients formulated by Peter Huttenlocher. Here, 60 percent of a patient's daily calorie intake now came in the form of MCT oil. Accordingly, a larger variety of meals were now available for sufferers, and so the ketogenic diet was born.

Ultimately, this was a significant discovery because it meant that patients could eat more carbohydrates and proteins, which lead to the possibility of a varied diet. And now we have the history behind the diet, let's look at it more **closely**.

Science of the Ketogenic Diet

Ketosis

The most important point to understand is that the ketogenic diet is a low carbohydrate, high fat diet. The intention behind it is for your body to produce ketones as a source of energy. This happens when your body transitions into a state called ketosis. This is achieved by eating fewer carbs (5% to 10%), more fat (60% to 75%) and moderate protein (15% to 30%).

Normally, your bodies process the carbohydrate we eat on an average balanced diet by turning it into glucose for energy. When ketosis is reached, your body begins to use the ketones produced from the transfer of fat to energy. If ketosis is maintained, your body can enter a metabolic state where it will continue to burn these ketones. Ketosis is not a foreign process for your body. It happens naturally when your glucose levels are lowThis process also helps improve your body's resistance to insulin and is an excellent choice for diabetics. We mentioned ketones, but what exactly are they? When our body breaks down fat for energy, certain byproducts are produced. These are known as ketone bodies or ketones for short. This process works as follows:

- ✓ When your body doesn't have enough glucose, your glycogen levels eventually run out.
- ✓ Your body now begins to burn fuel differently since the glycogen stores have now depleted. It does this by using fat to fuel itself.
- ✓ Your liver will start to produce ketones that fuel your body.
- ✓ When your body reaches this state, you are now under ketosis.

This process produces three ketone bodies we discussed earlier on:

- ✓ β-hydroxybutyrate
- ✓ acetoacetate
- ✓ acetone

Your metabolism is happy burning carbohydrates for fuel. Simple sugars from bread, rice and candy are broken down with little thought or energy, providing you with enough fuel to get through the day. When provided steady sources of carbohydrate throughout the day, things run smoothly. The problem is, unless you are giving your body only what it needs for carbohydrates, the rest of those simple sugars will be stored as fat to use later, perhaps if you miss a meal. Weight gain happens when you consistently eat more than your body needs to survive. Physiologically speaking, this is necessary, so you don't keel over between meals, but these days, inactivity plus huge portions mean you will keep storing fuel you don't intend to burn—you gain weight.

When you do not have a source of steady carbohydrates during the day, your metabolism shifts to pull fat from your stores, and burn it for energy. This fat-burning process is called ketosis, and the byproduct of this is ketones. Ketosis is the body's natural back up to burning carbohydrates as a matter of survival. As you could imagine, ketosis helps you lose weight because you are constantly burning fat for fuel instead of burning carbs as they come into your system. The problem is, it takes a bit of time to enter ketosis, and as soon as you eat carbohydrates, your body goes back to burning sugars. The good news is that you can build your diets around proteins and fats instead of carbohydrates to mimic carbohydrate starvation to push your body into ketosis.

While everyone will be a little bit different, the threshold of carbohydrates is about 50–60 grams per day, and about 10–15 grams per meal, before you exit ketosis. To put this into perspective, 15 grams is equal to a small slice of bread, which is not allowed on the ketogenic diet. To make the most of meals, most of these carbs will be in sources like vegetables with low carb content. The basic ketogenic meal is a combination of proteins like chicken and fish, with a large side of non-starchy vegetables like salad and zucchini. Fats can be used without real restriction too, so healthy fats like olive oil and avocado can be used to make up for the calories not taken up by carbohydrate-rich starches like rice and potato.

The primary goal of maintaining ketosis on the ketogenic diet is to force your body into a metabolic state. You do not want to do this through starvation, but rather through the starvation of carbohydrates. Our bodies are very adaptable, so when you switch your diet by loading it with fats instead of carbs, you burn ketones as an energy source. When you get to burning off optimal ketone levels, you then can lose weight faster and experience the physical and mental performance benefits the ketogenic diet has to offer.

The Process of Ketosis

A form of acidosis, ketosis disrupts the pH balance in your body due to the presence of more ketones in the blood. Ketones are a byproduct of your fat metabolism that are released when fat is broken down into an energy source. Metabolism on ketosis is when blood sugars are not readily available to your body as a source of energy, your body switches gears and starts to break down fat instead. When the ketones are broken down into glucose and released into your bloodstream, this is the start of ketosis. Produced in the liver, ketones can be utilized for other metabolic processes in your body. Getting to the point that you reach ketosis may seem complicated to those that are new to the keto diet. But overall, it is a straightforward process:

- ✓ Restrict carbs: Many people focus only on their intake of net carbs when they should be limiting total carbs. Try your best to stay below 20g of net carbs and 35g of total carbs.
- ✓ Restrict protein consumption: There are many folks who switch to the ketogenic diet from other diets and totally space off limiting their intake of protein. Eating too much protein can lead to drastically low levels of ketones, limiting ketosis. For sustained weight loss, you want to eat around 0.6–0.8 grams per pound to achieve that lean body mass you desire.
- ✓ Don't fret over fat: Fat is the primary source of energy on the keto diet, so you need to make it a priority to fuel your body with enough of it. Despite popular

belief, you are going to lose less weight if you starve yourself, no matter what diet you are on, so avoid this always.

✓ Drink water: When you first begin the keto diet, make it a goal to drink a gallon of water per day. This sounds like a lot, but you must stay hydrated to regulate your bodily functions and control your levels of hunger.

✓ Quit with the snacks: You can lose weight much easier when your body doesn't undergo multiple spikes in insulin throughout the day. Snacking for no reason can stall your weight loss achievements.

✓ Fast: Fasting is a good tool to help boost your ketone levels.

  o Skip a meal: Skipping a meal induces fasting. You can decide what meal to skip.

  o Limit your intake of food to a 4-7 hours window and leave the remaining time to fast.

  o 24-48-hour cleanses are when you do not eat for 1-2 days and experience extended fasting periods.

✓ Incorporate exercise: Exercise is a healthy habit for everyone. If you want to get the most out of undergoing the ketogenic diet, add 20-30 minutes to your regular exercise routine each day. Even an extra walk can help regulate blood sugar and promote more weight loss.

✓ Begin supplementing: This is not always needed, but it can help you get the best out of the keto diet.

There are several resources that you will come across in your hunt for achieving optimal ketosis. I recommend putting all those articles to the side because the most effective ketosis can be achieved easily through diet and nutrition. There is no magic pill, shortcut, or gimmick that will ultimately help you accomplish it. There is one method of measuring your ketosis levels that involves you urinating on a strip of paper, but these can be inaccurate and can cost a lot of money. Instead, know the physical symptoms that will naturally tell you that you are on the right track:

- ✓ Increased urination: The keto diet is a natural diuretic that increases acetoacetate, a ketone body that is excreted through the process of urinating.
- ✓ Dry mouth: Thanks to having to urinate more often, this can lead to dry mouth and being thirsty. This is another reason to drink lots of water so that you replenish your electrolytes effectively.
- ✓ Bad breath: A ketone body known as acetone is excreted into our mouth which affects the smell of our breath. It tends to smell like ripe fruit, sometimes even as potent as nail polish remover. This is temporary and goes away over time.
- ✓ Reduced hunger and increased energy: After you get past the "keto flu" stage, you will experience higher energy levels, a clear state of mind and will be hungry less often.
- ✓ Keto flu: This type of flu is a common phenomenon for newbies on the ketogenic diet, but thankfully it goes away after just a few days. You might experience mild discomfort in the form of cramps, nausea, headaches and fatigue.
- ✓ The following food wheel gives you an idea of the five main food groups and should serve as a helpful starting point for selecting the right foods for ketosis.

Ketoacidosis

There is often a lot of confusion when it comes to the difference between ketosis and ketoacidosis. Ketoacidosis happens in individuals who are diabetic and is often a complication of type 1 diabetics. It results from high levels of ketones in blood sugars, which can be life-threatening. This can make the blood too acidic, which has the potential to change the overall function of vital internal organs. This is not to be confused with the process of ketosis on the ketogenic diet.

Know Your Macros!

Macros is the abbreviation for the term macronutrients or the "big 3", comprising carbohydrates, protein and fats. You can use the macro calculator for figuring out what your personal daily needs should be. Fats are 10% anti-ketogenic and 90% ketogenic, thanks to the tiny bit of glucose that is released as our bodies convert the triglycerides. Proteins are 58% anti-ketogenic and 45% ketogenic because insulin levels are risen from half of the proteins we ingest that are converted to glucose. Carbs are 100% anti-ketogenic since they are responsible for the rise in insulin and blood glucose levels. What does this mean? Simply that carbs and protein hurt the act of trying to get into the state of ketosis. So, it is vital to learn how they are being converted to energy, which is through metabolic pathways after being ingested as nutrients.

Your Body on the Ketogenic Diet

With all this new information, you may be wondering how you will physically be feeling when you first start undergoing the keto transformation. Your body is more than likely accustomed to a simple routine of breaking down the carbohydrates you consume into energy. Your body has already built up the enzymes it needs to process these carbs, which means they are by no means used to dealing with the breaking down and storage of fats. This means that your body is having to deal with and become used to a lack of glucose but an increase in fat consumption, which means it must produce a whole new supply of enzymes. Once your body starts to become used to the state of ketosis, you will naturally shift to utilize what glucose you have left in storage. Therefore, your muscles will have a depleted supply of glycogen, which can mean lethargy and a lack of overall energy.

During the first week of undergoing the keto diet, many people report being dizzy, easily aggravated and headaches. This is because your electrolytes are flushed from your system. Another reason is to drink lots of water and keep up with your sodium intake: salt helps you to retain water, which replenishes your electrolytes.

Side Effects of the Ketogenic Diet

The keto flu

This type of flu is a common phenomenon for newbies on the ketogenic diet, but thankfully it goes away just after a few days. You might also experience mild discomfort in the form of cramps, nausea, headaches and fatigue.

The keto flu occurs due to two main reasons:

1. You are going to the bathroom more often to urinate, which means you are losing electrolytes and water within the body. You can combat this easily by drinking a bouillon cube in water.

2. Your body is in a phase of total transition. You are used to processing a higher intake of carbohydrates. Your body needs a bit of time to create the enzymes needed to process a higher intake of fat. Therefore, you may feel low on energy. It is best to gradually decrease your intake of carbs and not go cold turkey.

Once you increase your water consumption and replace electrolytes, you will find that the symptoms of the keto flu decrease or totally diminish. For a person that is beginning the transition to the ketogenic diet, it is recommended to eat less than 15 grams of carbs a day and decrease this amount over time. All good things in life tend to have a bad side. Luckily, these risks are not near as negative as ones you have the chance to experience on other diets.

✓ **Fatigue and irritability** – Even though raised ketone levels can drastically improve a few areas regarding your physical quality of life, they are also directly related to feeling tired and having to work harder during physical activities.

- ✓ **"Brain fog"** – If you stay on the ketogenic diet long term, there is going to be a major shifting when it comes to the metabolic areas of your body. This can make you moody and somewhat sluggish, which can make you not able to think clearly or adequately focus. Ensure that you are reducing your levels of carb intake at steady levels, not all at once.

- ✓ **Lipids may change** – Even though fats on the ketogenic diet are welcomed, if you consume large amounts of saturated fats, your cholesterol levels will begin to increase. Make sure you are consuming healthy fats.

- ✓ **Micronutrient deficiencies** – Diets that consist of low-carb foods are more than likely lacking in essential nutrients, such as magnesium, potassium and iron. You might want to strongly consider finding a high-quality multivitamin to take daily.

- ✓ **Developing ketoacidosis** – If your ketone levels become too out of whack, it may lead to this condition. pH levels within your blood decrease, creating an environment that is high in acidity, which can be threatening for those with diabetes.

- ✓ **Muscle loss** – As you consume less energy, your body leans on the help of other tissues as a source of fuel. If you work out heavily while on a diet like the ketogenic diet, there is the potential for major muscle loss.

Benefits of the Ketogenic Diet

All types of low-carb diets have been on the table of controversy for quite a few years. It has been said that diets high in fat content can raise cholesterol levels through the roof, causing heart disease and other bad body ailments. But research has shown that amongst other diets, low-carb ones win the race. They are not only a great substitute when trying to lose weight, but they even have other great health benefits, even reducing cholesterol levels. Here are some ways that the Ketogenic Diet can produce some good things in your life!

The main component that is largely working in your body during your time on the ketogenic diet is the process of ketosis. Creating this metabolic state has been proven to have drastically positive effects, even if only on the diet for a short time. Here are some grand benefits of ketosis itself first!

- ✓ Increases our body's capabilities to use fats as a source of fuel.
- ✓ Ketosis has a protein-sparing effect, which means our bodies prefer utilizing ketones as opposed to glucose.
- ✓ Lowers levels of insulin within our bodies, which contains a lipolysis-blocking effect, which reduces the utilization of fatty acids as a source of energy. When insulin levels are lowered, growth hormones and other growth factors can then be released without an issue.
- ✓ Suppresses hunger – Naturally, many diets require you to eat less than your body is used to. Because of this, never-ending hunger pains always seem to strike and at the worst times. This is the main reason people tend to feel miserable while on any diet plan. Diets that are low in carb intake are great because it automatically reduces your appetite. Those who cut carbs and consume more proteins and fat actually eat *fewer* calories.
- ✓ More potential for weight loss – People who stick within the means of low-carb diets lose weight at a much faster rate than those who within the means of a low-carb diet. Diets low in carbohydrates tend to help in the reduction of excess water in our bodies, which can add on the pounds. The ketogenic diet reduces insulin levels too, meaning the kidneys are shedding excess sodium that can lead to retaining extra weight.
- ✓ Reduction of triglycerides – This is a fancy name for fat molecules. These little boogers contribute to ailments such as heart disease. When people reduce the consumption of carbs, there is quite a lessening of triglycerides building up in our bodies.

- ✓ Increase of good cholesterol levels – HDL is the kind of cholesterol you *want* to have. The ketogenic diet helps with raising HDL levels because of the consumption of fats. There are major bodily improvements when the levels of good and bad cholesterol start to shift.

- ✓ Reduces blood sugar and insulin levels – When we consume carbs, they are broken into simple sugars by our digestive system. They then go into our bloodstreams and elevate blood sugar levels. High sugars can be toxic, which is why insulin exists. There are many people who have a type of diabetes not only because of bloodlines and genetics, but because they have not eaten the best for quite a bit of their life. Their bodies no longer recognize insulin when it is attempting to help lower blood sugar levels. With the ketogenic diet, it has been seen that blood sugar and insulin levels come way down.

- ✓ Reduction in blood pressure – Diets that are low in carbohydrates are effective in reducing blood pressure levels, which can assist us in living longer. When blood pressure is high, we are at greater risks of developing hypertension and other ailments.

- ✓ Natural treatment for cancer – Properly regulating your body's metabolic functions has been proven to be a great step in reducing and even treating cancer. Reducing or totally removing carbs from your diet can help in the deletion of energy from cancerous cells and stop them from spreading.

- ✓ Effective in treating metabolic syndrome – This syndrome is actually a serious medical condition that is associated with heart disease and diabetes. There are several symptoms:
  - ✓ Low levels of HDL
  - ✓ High triglyceride levels
  - ✓ Raised fasting blood sugar levels
  - ✓ Elevated blood pressure
  - ✓ Abdominal obesity

✓ Therapy for some brain disorders – There are certain areas of our brains that strictly run on glucose as a fuel. This is the reason behind why our livers produce it from protein if we do not consume carbs. There are bigger portions of our brains, however, that burn through ketones. Think back to Charlie Abraham, who was mentioned earlier in this chapter. In studies, more than half of children who utilized the ketogenic diet had a 50% reduction in seizures.

Foods to Avoid

✓ Grains: Rice, corn, oats, wheat, barley, etc. Pasta, bread, cookies, crackers, etc.
✓ Factory-farmed fish and pork
✓ Processed foods
✓ Artificial sweeteners
✓ Refined fats and oils
✓ Foods that are "low-fat," "low-carb" or "zero-carb"
✓ Milk
✓ Alcoholic and sweet beverages
✓ Soy products

Foods to Eat

Any diet can be challenging when you are not aware of what to eat and what not to eat. Thankfully, you have an entire list of ketogenic must and must-not eats to ensure you stay on the right track!

Grass-Fed and Wild Animal Sources	Healthy Fats	Non-Starchy veggies	Fruits	Beverages and Condiments
Beef	**Saturated**	**Leafy greens**	Avocado	Water
Lamb				Black coffee
Goat	Coconut oil	Radicchio	**Berries** mulberries	Tea
Venison	Butter	Endive	cranberries	Pork rinds
Fish and seafood	Ghee	Chives	raspberries	Mayo
Pork	Goose fat	Chard	strawberries	Mustard
Poultry	Duck fat	Lettuce	blueberries	Pesto
Eggs	Chicken fat	Spinach	blackberries	Bone Broth
Gelatin	Tallow	Bok choy		Pickles and other
Ghee	Lard	Swiss chard	Sugar snap peas	fermented eats
Liver, heart,			Artichokes	Spices
kidneys, and	**Monounsaturated**	**Cruciferous**	Water chestnuts	Lemon/lime juice &
other organ		**vegetables**	Sea vegetables	zest
meats	Olive oil			Whey protein
	Macadamia oil	Radishes	**Root veggies**	
Nuts & Seeds	Avocado oil	Kohlrabi	pumpkin	
Sunflower seeds		Dark leaf kale	winter squash	
Pecans	**Polyunsaturated**	Celery	mushrooms	
Almonds		Asparagus	Cabbage	
Walnuts	Fatty fish and seafood	Cucumber	Cauliflower	
Hazelnuts		Summer squash	Broccoli	
Macadamia nuts		(spaghetti squash,	Fennel	
		zucchini)	Brussels sprouts	
		Bamboo shoots		

Understanding Fats

Since fats make up a large and important portion of your keto diet, they are vital for staying healthy and in shape. But it is not just consuming fat this is crucial, but choosing the right fats is important as well! There can be a lot of confusion as to what fats are good, bad, and those which should be avoided when cooking with your Instant Pot. Here we will break down those good and bad fats.

Good Fats

The "good guy" fats that are a go in your diet are split up into four different categories:

1.   Saturated Fats
2.   Monounsaturated fats (MUFAs)
3.   Polyunsaturated fats (PUFAs)
4.   Trans fats (naturally occurring)

When it boils down to "what types of aspects are in what fats," you must remember that all fats in the world are created by a mixture of all the above types of fat but are categorized by which one is the most dominant. Here, we will break down each type of fat when it comes to consuming foods with your Instant Pot. This will help you to easily see them when you are making decisions about what to fuel your body and mind with.

Saturated Fats

These fats had a bad reputation for many years. They were viewed as terrible for the health of your heart and we were taught to avoid them.

However, since then there have been various studies that prove this wrong by showing no significant link between saturated fats and the risk of heart disease. We have been consuming saturated fats for *thousands* of years. Considering this new information, there is a plethora of great benefits that come along with the inclusion of healthy saturated fats in your daily diet.

Several saturated fats include something we call "medium-chain triglycerides (MCTs)," which are found in items like coconut oil and small amounts of butter and palm oil. MCT can be digested simply and easily in the body. When we eat these MCT's, they pass through the liver and are utilized automatically as an energy source! This means they are superb in your diet if you want to lose weight or boost your physical performance.

Health benefits of saturated fats:

- ✓ Increase in the function of the immune system
- ✓ Better cholesterol levels, both HDL and LDL
- ✓ Better HDL to LDL cholesterol ratio
- ✓ Improved maintenance of bone density
- ✓ Rise of HDL (good) cholesterol to prevent LDL within the arteries
- ✓ Promotes the creation of hormones like cortisol and testosterone, which are important for various reasons

Best sources of saturated fats:

- ✓ Butter
- ✓ Cocoa butter
- ✓ Coconut oil
- ✓ Cream
- ✓ Eggs
- ✓ Lard
- ✓ Palm oil
- ✓ Red meat

Monounsaturated Fats

Unlike saturated fats, monounsaturated fatty acids (MUFAs) have been a graciously accepted "good fat" for a long time. There have been a variety of studies that have directly linked MUFA's with benefits such as insulin resistance and good cholesterol levels.

Health benefits of MUFAs:

- ✓ Better levels of HDL cholesterol
- ✓ Decrease in blood pressure
- ✓ Decreased risk of developing heart disease
- ✓ Decrease in belly fat
- ✓ Decrease in insulin resistance

Best sources of MUFAs to eat:

- ✓ Avocados and avocado oil
- ✓ Extra virgin olive oil
- ✓ Goose fat
- ✓ Lard and bacon fat
- ✓ Macadamia nut oil

Polyunsaturated Fats

When it comes to consuming polyunsaturated fatty acids (PUFAs), it boils most importantly down to the type. When PUFAs are heated up, they can create free radicals, which are harmful to the body and responsible in the increase of inflammation and have been shown to increase the risk of developing cancer and heart disease. In other words, the majority of PUFAs should be eaten in cold forms and should never be utilized for cooking.

PUFAs can be found in processed oils and other extremely healthy sources. Eating the correct kinds of PUFAs can give you benefits, especially when you incorporate them into your diet. They include Omega 3's and Omega 6's, which are essential to feeling great!

The amount of PUFA's that you eat is extremely crucial. The ratio of omega 3 to omega 6 should be around 1:1. But most of Western diets consume a ratio of 1:30.

Health benefits of PUFAs:

When you consume a good balance of omega 3 and omega 6, you greatly reduce the risk of developing the following:

✓ Autoimmune disorders and other inflammatory diseases

✓ Heart disease

✓ Intake of PUFAs may even help improve symptoms of depression and help those with ADHD, which are more benefits associated with a keto diet.

✓ Stroke

Best sources of PUFA's to eat:

✓ Avocado oil

✓ Chia seeds

✓ Extra virgin olive oil

✓ Fatty fish and fish oil

✓ Flaxseeds and flaxseed oil

✓ Nut oils

✓ Sesame oil

✓ Walnuts

Trans Fats

You are probably questioning the author's intelligence seeing trans fats under the "good" fats category. But it does have a right to be in this section! Yes, the majority of trans fats are wildly unhealthy and can be very harmful to the human body, there *is* a type of trans fat, known as *vaccenic acid*, that is good for you! It is naturally found in foods like grass-fed meats and dairy products.

Health benefits of vaccenic acid can include:

✓ Decreased risk of developing diabetes and obesity

✓ Decreased risk of developing heart disease

✓ Protection against developing cancer

Best sources of healthy and natural trans fats to eat:

✓ Dairy fats such as butter and yogurt

✓ Grass-fed animal products

Bad Fats

One of the positive aspects that attract many people to the keto diet is that they can consume lots of satisfying foods and healthy fats. But, lurking around the corner, there are also bad fats that you must keep an eye on. You want to get rid of and eliminate these pesky guys, so you don't damage your bodily health. One of the key things to remember is that the quality of the food genuinely matters.

Processed Trans and Polyunsaturated Fats

Processed trans fats are a common type of fat that many of you are familiar with. They have the capability of being wildly detrimental to your overall physical wellbeing.

Artificial trans fats are created during the production of food, which occurs when polyunsaturated fats are processed. Therefore, it's important to only choose PUFAs that are unprocessed that are not overheated or altered in any way. Not The processing of PUFAs creates free radicals that are harmful when consumed and they are made from oils that contain genetically modified seeds.

Risks of consuming trans fats include:
- ✓ Bad for the health of your gut
- ✓ Increased risk of developing cancer
- ✓ Increased risk of developing heart disease
- ✓ Lead cause of inflammatory health issues
- ✓ Decrease in the good HDL cholesterol and increase of bad LDL cholesterol

Examples of trans fats to *eliminate*:
- ✓ Hydrogenated and partially hydrogenated oils that are in processed products like cookies, crackers, margarine, and fast food
- ✓ Processed vegetable oils like cottonseed, sunflower, safflower, soybean, and canola oils

Steps to Success on the Ketogenic Diet

This chapter is full of fool-proof ways to keep yourself on track as your venture down the Instant Pot road.

✓ Hydration: This should be something you do daily already but consume 32 ounces of water within the first hour that you get out of bed in the morning and strive to drink up another 32-48 ounces before the noon hour. Drink at *least* half of your weight in ounces of water or close to your full body weight in ounces daily to keep your overall hydration at healthy levels.

✓ Practice intermittent fasting: Start reducing your carb intake a couple to a few days before getting down and dirty. Break your day down into two phases:

- o **Building phase:** Amount of time between first and last meal
- o **Cleaning phase:** Amount of time between last and first meal

Start with a 12-16-hour cleaning phase and an 8-12-hour building phase. Your body will adapt over time, which will enable you to move to a 4-6-hour building time paired with an 18-20-hour cleaning phase each day.

Eat lots of salt: We are reminded all the time to lower our consumption of sodium. When you undergo a low-carb diet, insulin levels decrease, and our kidneys excrete higher levels of sodium. This results in a lowering of our sodium/potassium ratio.

- o Add ¼ teaspoon of pink salt to glasses of water
- o Add kelp, nori or dulse to dishes
- o Be generous with amount of pink salt you add to food
- o Consume pumpkin seeds or macadamia nuts as a snack
- o Drink organic broth off and on throughout the day
- o Eat cucumber or celery; both have natural sodium

✓ Exercise on a regular basis: High-intensity exercise daily help to assist in activating glucose molecules known as GLUT-4 which are responsible for reciting information to various areas of the body back to the liver and muscle tissues. This receptor takes away sugar that is in the bloodstream and uses it as muscle and liver glycogen. Exercising on a regular basis doubles the levels of crucial proteins in both the muscles and liver.

✓ Work on improving mobility of bowels: Many people struggle with constipation issues. To help, consume fermented edibles, such as sauerkraut, coconut water, kimchi, etc. It is recommended to take extra supplements, such as magnesium. Drinking one green drink per day will also help to increase the levels of calcium, magnesium, and potassium in your system, all of which help aid constipation and promote healthy bowel movement.

✓ Don't eat too much protein: Even though consumption of proteins is recommended following a keto diet, some people do not know a proper balance and eat too much protein. Your body will change all those amino acids into glucose through the process known as gluconeogenesis if you eat too much protein. You will probably have to play with the amounts of protein you eat because some people need than others.

✓ Choose your carbs wisely: For a keto diet, it is best to consume at least some good types of carbohydrates, such as starchy veggies and fruits likes berries, apples or citrus. Combine them into a green smoothie for a great morning pick-me-up!

✓ Utilize mct oil: The usage of high-quality medium chain triglyceride (MCT) is crucial for replenishing your energy levels throughout the day. You can cook with this oil as well as add it to coffee, tea, green drinks, protein shakes and more!

✓ Keep stress to a minimum: The buildup of daily stress will inhibit our energy levels. If you are under constant chronic stress, then now may not be the time to undergo any form of diet, but rather a diet that concentrates on being anti-inflammatory and lower in carbs instead.

✓ Improve the quality of sleep: If you are not getting adequate amounts of rest, this is another aspect that can lead to a rise in stress hormones. Ensure that you are in a dark room that you feel comfortable in. It is recommended to get around 7-9 hours of sleep per night. The more stressed you are, the more sleep you need. Ensure that you are sleeping in a room that is no warmer than 65-70 degrees.

✓ Consume Ghee: Ghee is a great substitute for butter, if not a total replacement! It is highly recommended, and you can use it as normally as you utilize butter.

✓ Take omega-3's: It is important to consume or take Omega-3 vitamins. You should have higher levels of Omega 3's than Omega 6's in your diet. Eating all that oil will cause you harm if your Omega's are not properly balanced.

✓ Avoid alcohol: While this sounds like a bummer, the consumption of alcohol can put a stop to your weight loss. Which is worth it: that bottle of beer or being able to fit into those clothes you are hanging on to in hopes you will once again fit into them?

✓ Make lemon water your best friend: Not only is it tasty and refreshing, but lemon water helps to balance out your pH levels, which can create the perfect environment.

✓ Avoid "sugar-free" products: Even though it sounds better for you, try to avoid products that say "sugar-free" or "light" because these more than likely have more carbs than their original counterparts.

✓ Avoid low-fat: You should steer clear and not waste your precious time with anything that is low in fat. You need to have high percentages of fat in your diet in order to maintain an adequate and healthy balance. Otherwise, the protein you consume may be converted into sugars too.

✓ Get a food scale: This tool is important to have in your kitchen if you want total success. Being accurate is vital to the process of monitoring what you are fueling your body with. If you plan to track carbs and count calories, you really need to know what you are consuming. Make sure the scale you buy has a conversion button, an automatic shutoff, a tare function, as well as a removable plate.

✓ Know healthy alternatives to carbs: You will inevitably have cravings from time to time. There is something about fried chicken, rice, sauces, and more that make your mouth water. For ultimate satisfaction, it is a good idea to have alternatives and substitutes up your sleeve to combat. Try some of these alternatives!

- **Shirataki noodles** are low-carb, which makes them a perfect alternative when you have a hankering for pasta!

- **Cauliflower rice** can be used in the place of regular white or brown rice.

- **Spaghetti squash** can be creatively turned into noodles with the help of a spiralizer or simply with a fork. Awesome taste and less than half the carbs and calories.

- Use **heavy whipping cream** or **almond milk** in your coffee instead of that calorie-packed creamer.

- For those that love and constantly crave bread, there are many low-carb options, such as **low-carb bread and tortillas**!

- You will find that when your sweet tooth needs a bit of love that making shakes or smoothies with the help of **protein powder.** There are tons of flavors that can be easily mixed into batters, snacks, and much more! Plus, it gives you a nice boost of protein without sacrificing all the hard work you have put into eating a keto diet.

INSTANT POT 101

REVOLUTIONARY...

The Instant Pot is the brand name for a programmable countertop multi-cooker. Specifically, the device itself is a single countertop appliance that can perform multiple functions. The instant pot can replace the following:

- ✓ Slow Cooker
- ✓ Pressure Cooker
- ✓ Rice Cooker
- ✓ Steamer
- ✓ Sauté/Browning Pan
- ✓ Yogurt Maker
- ✓ Warming Pan

Did you forget to thaw out something for dinner? No problem—the Instant Pot can handle it! The instant pot can cook baked potatoes in minutes and come out so fluffy on the inside too – tasty! Also, it can cook veggies in about five minutes while also preserving their nutrients. It's also a slow cooker too. Did you catch that—it's a slow cooker that doesn't boil over! When it's finished slow cooking, it goes to the warm setting. Your food doesn't continue to cook, instead the instant pot keeps it warm! This single appliance has changed the way I cook! Most days, I use the Slow Cooker or Instant Pot features. Because of this, I spend less time in the kitchen and more time doing the things I love. My grocery basket is now filled with vegetables because the instant pot perfectly cooks them while not destroying any of their nutrients.

Once a week, I cook up a batch of hardboiled eggs for a quick breakfast when I must take my grandchildren to school early in the morning. The sauté/browning feature means that I can sauté veggies and brown meat in a single pot before setting the slow cooker. I occasionally toss things in the pot and set it to the warming feature. It will warm up my food and keep it warm for hours! You can put frozen soup into the pot in the morning, set it on Warm, and have perfectly heated soup for dinner ten hours later. This single appliance has made cooking faster and more convenient (Even my husband has taken to using it!). I love that I can cook steel-cut oats for breakfast in a fraction of the time it would take on the stovetop, make rice to go with a last-minute stir-fry is in minutes, and slow-cook a stew. In fact, it's even taken the place of my slow cooker, which has since been moved out of the kitchen.

Is the Instant Pot Safe?

You might be wondering why I would want an instant pot. Don't they occasionally explode and leave sweet potatoes on the ceiling? Well, this is not your grandmother's instant pot! Modern instant pots, or pressure cookers, have several safety features that are electronically controlled. It is impossible to open the lid of one until the pressure has been released either naturally or manually—so burning hazards are minimized! Rest assured, modern day electric pressure cookers like the Instant Pot are quiet, safe and easy to use. They have 10 UL Certified proven safety mechanisms to prevent most potential issues. This means that they are very safe to use in your kitchen provided you use your common sense—for example, be careful with water spillages and keep your instant pot away from children, pets and vulnerable people.

Don't pre-heat the cooker!

I got into the habit of preheating the base of the pressure cooker on a low flame to give me time to slice onions or peel garlic cloves while the cooker was pre-heating. But, on induction, I kept getting burned olive oil and charred onions. Don't pre-heat your cooker on induction because the cooking surface is hot and ready to sauté in 15 seconds!

Don't bring the cooker to pressure on high heat!

Following the old standby advice about bringing the cooker to pressure on high heat, several obvious things will happen: the cooker reaches pressure at break-neck speed (about 4 minutes), tomato sauces carbonize and bond to the base of the cooker and the food comes out disappointingly under-done.

Don't walk away from a full cooker after you've adjusted the heat!

Although the cooker may have reached the correct pressure, the sides are still at a lower temperature than the hot aluminum-disk-clad base. Walking away from the cooker once it has cooled will cause the internal pressure to quickly fall because the heat generated from the base is not enough to keep the food inside boiling and maintaining pressure and heat up the rest of the cooker or food inside of it.

Do's!

✓ **DO** bring the pressure cooker to pressure on medium heat or tack on a few minutes to the cooking time to compensate for the lower pressure-cooking temperature and shorter time to pressure.

✓ **DO** hang around to make heat adjustments for the first 5 minutes of pressure for very full or very wide cookers.

✓ **DO** use the induction burner's timer feature to set the pressure-cooking time so the burner turns itself off automatically when time is up!

✓ **DO** slice the aromatics first, and then turn on the induction burner just before tossing oil or aromatics to sauté.

INSTANT POT FAQS

Is the instant pot the same as a pressure cooker?

Absolutely! The Instant Pot is currently one of the most popular electric pressure cooker brands. It is a multi-functional cooker that has some extra functions compared to traditional stove-top pressure cookers – it is also incredibly faster too!

Instapot or instant pot?

Many people call the Instant Pot a pressure cooker, InstaPot, IP or IPPY. The correct name is Instant Pot but call it whatever you like. In fact, some users even name their cookers. I call mine Toby after my childhood dog. In fact, you can also buy swanky covers to put on it too.

Is it easy to cook with an instant pot?

There's a learning curve to cook with pressure cookers. But no worries! Once you're familiar with it, you will find the cooking relatively easy.

Does the instant pot really speed up the cooking process?

Cooking in any pressure cooker is almost always faster. It may not be noticeable for some foods like broccoli or shrimps. However, tender and juicy pulled pork can be done in under 90 minutes, when it usually takes 2 – 4 hours to make in the oven.

Are there disadvantages cooking in the instant pot?

One disadvantage cooking with any pressure cooker is that you can't inspect, taste or adjust the food along the way. That's why it's essential to follow recipes with accurate cooking times (like those recipes in this book).

Can I use the instant pot for pressure frying?

Please don't attempt to pressure fry in any electric pressure cookers. The splattering oil may melt the gasket. KFC uses a commercial pressure fryer (modern ones operate at 5 PSI) specially made to fry chickens. The Chicken recipes in this book is probably as close as it gets.

How to do a quick release?

After the cooking cycle ends, carefully move the venting knob from sealing position to venting position. This rapidly releases the pressure in the pressure cooker. This usually takes a few minutes. Wait until the floating valve (metal pin) completely drops before opening the lid.

How to do a natural release?

After the cooking cycle ends, wait until the floating valve (metal pin) completely drops before opening the lid. Always turn the venting knob from sealing position to venting position. This ensures all the pressure is released before opening the lid. It usually takes 10 – 25 minutes. In these recipes, you may see "15 mins Natural Release" – this means after the cooking cycle ends, wait 15 minutes before turning the venting knob to manually release the remaining pressure.

Instant Pot
RECIPES

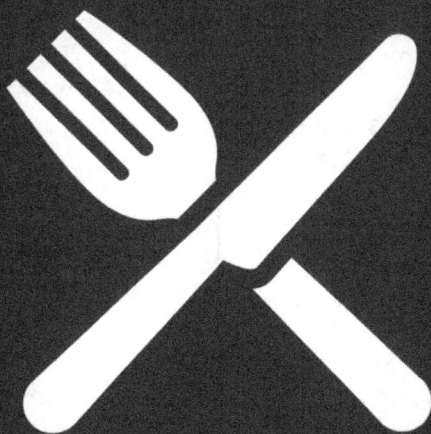

Egg Sandwich

What's inside:

- ✓ Sesame seeds (.5 Tbsp.)
- ✓ Peeled and pitted avocado (1)
- ✓ Rinsed lettuce leaves (2)
- ✓ Sliced red onion (.5)
- ✓ Whole egg (1)

How to make:

1. Take out your Instant Pot and add a cup of water in. then add the egg to the middle and close up the lid.
2. Check the steam valve and have it set to Sealing. Then press the Manual button and let these cook.
3. After 5 minutes, you can do a quick pressure release.
4. When the pressure is gone, open the lid, take the egg out, and then peel the egg. Slice this egg up and set aside.
5. Now you can assemble your burgers. Place the egg, onion, and lettuce leaves in between your avocado slices.
6. Sprinkle some pepper and salt on top and then garnish with some sesame seeds before serving.

Nutritional information:

Calories: 478
Carbs: 19.1g
Protein: 13.9g
Fat: 41.2g

Spicy Egg Skillet

What's inside:

- ✓ Chopped jalapeno peppers (4)
- ✓ Eggs (4)
- ✓ Grated cauliflower (1 head)
- ✓ Minced garlic cloves (#)
- ✓ Olive oil (1 Tbsp.)

How to make:

1. Turn on your Instant Pot and get it warmed up. Then add in the oil and the garlic and stir these around for a minute.
2. Add in the cauliflower and season with some pepper and salt. Then pour in half a cup of water, making sure to spread it out evenly on the bottom of your inner pot.
3. Make four little wells in your cauliflower and crack an egg into each one. Top with the jalapeno peppers.
4. Close the lid and check that the steam valve is working right. Press the Manual button and let these cook.
5. After six minutes, release the pressure and serve.

Nutritional information:

Calories: 113
Carbs: 6.2g
Protein: 4.6g
Fat: 9.5g

Salmon and Avocado Breakfast Meal

What's inside:

- ✓ Juice from one lemon
- ✓ Olive oil (2 Tbsp.)
- ✓ Pitted avocado (1)
- ✓ Salt and pepper
- ✓ Wild salmon fillets (2 oz.)

How to make:

1. Take your steamer basket and place it into your prepared Instant Pot. Add in a bit of water.
2. Take the salmon fillets and season them with some pepper and salt to your liking. Then take these prepared salmon fillets and add them on top of the steamer basket.
3. Close the lid of the Instant Pot and press the Steam button. Let the salmon cook.
4. After ten minutes, you can take the salmon out of the Instant pot. Place the salmon into a bowl and flake it.
5. Stir in the lemon juice and olive oil and season some more if you want with pepper and salt.
6. Spoon the prepared fish into the hollowed out portions of the avocado before serving.

Nutritional information

Calories: 661
Carbs: 27.8g
Protein: 13.5g
Fat: 68.2g

Basil Omelet

What's inside:

- ✓ Chopped basil leaves (1 c.)
- ✓ Pepper and salt
- ✓ Coconut milk (.25 c.)
- ✓ Beaten eggs 6)
- ✓ Olive oil (2 Tbsp.)

How to make:

1. Take out a mixing bowl and combine together all the ingredients, leaving out the basil leaves.
2. Place the basil into the inner pot of your Instant Pot and pour your eggs over these.
3. Put the lid on top of the Instant Pot and press the "Slow Cooker" function to cook.
4. After four hours, the dish is done. Let the steam out and allow the dish to cool before serving.

Nutritional information

Calories: 195
Carbs: 2.3g
Protein: 9.4g
Fat: 16.5g

Keto Porridge

What's inside:

- ✓ Salt
- ✓ Coconut oil (2 Tbsp.)
- ✓ Coconut cream (5 Tbsp.)
- ✓ Sesame seeds (1 Tbsp.)
  Beaten eggs (2)

How to make:

1. Take out a mixing bowl and combine the five ingredients above. Pour this into your prepared Instant Pot.
2. Close the lid on the Instant Pot and then press your Slow Cooker function on the pot.
3. After 4 hours, you can slowly release the pressure and let the porridge cool down before you enjoy.

Nutritional information:

Calories: 691
Carbs: 8g
Fat: 22.9g
Fat: 77.5g

Western Omelet

What's inside:

- ✓ Coconut milk (.25 c.)
- ✓ Beaten eggs (6)
- ✓ Chopped bell pepper (.5)
- ✓ Chopped yellow onion (1)
- ✓ Ground beef (.5 c.)

How to make:

1. Add your ground beef into the Instant Pot and warm it up. Cook this for a few minutes to make the beef lightly brown before adding in the bell pepper and onion.
2. Turn the Instant Pot off after these ingredients have time to heat up a bit and set aside.
3. In a bowl, mix together the coconut milk and eggs until they are well combined. Pour this mixture over the beef in the Instant Pot and then close the lid.
4. Turn this onto the Slow Cooker function. This mixture needs to cook for four hours before serving.

Nutritional information:

Calories: 244
Carbs: 2.7g
Protein: 10.6g
Fat: 20.5g

Healthy Morning Muffins

What's inside:

- ✓ Avocado slices (4)
- ✓ Pepper and salt
- ✓ Whole egg (4)
- ✓ Uncured bacon (4 strips)
- ✓ Olive oil (1 Tbsp.)

How to make:

1. Take out the Instant Pot and place a steam rick inside. Pour in about a cup of water to the bottom.
2. Take out four muffin cups and grease them with some oil. Place a strip into each of these prepared muffin cups.
3. Crack an egg over your bacon strips and then season wit some pepper and salt before adding these muffin cups into that steam rack from before.
4. Close the lid on the Instant Pot and press the Steam function to start cooking the muffins.
5. After 8 minutes, do a quick release of the pressure to let all the steam out. Garnish these muffins with some avocado slices and enjoy.

Nutritional information:

Calories: 501
Carbs: 19.5g
Protein: 13.7g
Fat: 43.9g

Blackberry Egg Cake

What's inside:

- ✓ Zest from half an orange
- ✓ Blackberries (.5 c.)
- ✓ Coconut flour (3 Tbsp.)
- ✓ Coconut oil (1 Tbsp.)
- ✓ Eggs (5)

How to make:

1. Take your steam rack and add it to the Instant Pot with a cup of water to heat up.
2. In a bowl, combine the coconut flour, coconut oil, and eggs together until well combined. Season with just a bit of salt.
3. Add the orange zest and the blackberries in as well before pouring this whole mixture into muffin cups.
4. Place the muffin cups on a steam rack in the Instant Pot and then close up the lid.
5. Press the Steam function when you are ready to cook. This meal needs to cook for 8 minutes.
6. When this time is done, do a quick pressure release and then allow the cake time to cool down before you serve.

Nutritional information:

Calories: 172
Carbs: 11.4g
Protein: 5.6g
Fat: 16.9g

Monkey Bread

What's inside:

- ✓ Brown sugar (.5 c.)
- ✓ Butter (.5 stick)
- ✓ Buttered and premade biscuits (1 can)
- ✓ Cinnamon (1.5 tsp.)
- ✓ Sugar (.5 c.)

How to make:

1. Take out a big bowl and add the cinnamon and sugar. Slice up four of the biscuits to make four pieces each. Coat these with the sugar mixture and place into a mini loaf pan.
2. Repeat this process to fill up another pan as well.
3. Add the brown sugar and the butter into a bowl that is safe for the microwave and then heat it up for 45 seconds. When it is melted well, stir it around with a fork.
4. Divide this sauce between your two prepared loaf pans.
5. Add in a cup of water to the Instant Pot and then place a trivet inside. Place both of the loaf pans in the Instant Pot.
6. Cover these pans with some foil before closing the lid nice and tight on it all.
7. You can select "Manually High Pressure" to get this stared. After 21 minutes, allow the pressure to release naturally for about five minutes, then you can do the quick pressure release to finish up.
8. Remove the lid slowly and take the Monkey Bread out of the pot before serving.

Nutritional information

Calories: 215
Carbs: 10g
Protein: 1g
Fat: 13g

Breakfast Cobbler

What's inside:

- ✓ Granola (1 c.)
- ✓ Cinnamon (.5 tsp.)
- ✓ Butter (3 Tbsp.)
- ✓ Honey 2 Tbsp.)
- ✓ Diced apple (2)

How to make:

1. Place your diced apple into a stainless steel bowl that will fit into the Instant Pot. Add in the cinnamon, butter, and honey and stir to combine well.
2. Close the lid on the Instant Pot and select "Manually High Pressure." After the ten minutes are up, do a quick pressure release.
3. Use a slotted spoon to move the cooked fruit over. Add the granola to the liquid left in the Instant Pot.
4. Allow these ingredients to cook for a few minutes but stir on a regular basis.
5. After about five minutes are done, you can take the granola out of the Instant Pot and place it on the cooked fruit.
6. Serve this warm with some coconut whipped cream if you would like.

Nutritional information:

Calories: 385
Carbs: 12g
Protein: 1g
Fat: 15g

On the Go Egg Cups

What's inside:

- ✓ Pepper and salt
- ✓ Half and half (.25 c.)
- ✓ Grated cheddar cheese (.5 c.)
- ✓ Diced vegetables of choice (1 c.)
- ✓ Eggs (4)

How to make:

1. Take out some jars and grease them with butter or oil.
2. Take out a bowl and beat the eggs with the pepper, salt, half and half, cheese, and vegetables.
3. When that mixture is done, divide it between four half-pint, wide-mouth, heatproof jars. Place the lids on the jars, but don't tighten them.
4. Pour a few cups of water into the Instant Pot and add a trivet to the bottom. Add the egg jars to this trivet.
5. Lock the lid in place on the pot and select Manual. Have the pressure at a high setting.
6. After 5 minutes, the dish is done and you can use the quick release method to get rid of all the steam.
7. Take the lids from the jars and then top these with the cheese of your choice.
8. You can then add these to an air fryer for a few minutes to get the cheese melted before serving.

Nutritional information:

Calories: 239
Carbs: 7g
Protein: 15g
Fat: 17g

Cheese Frittata

What's inside:

- ✓ Eggs (4)
- ✓ Half and half (1 c.)
- ✓ Chopped green chills (1 can)
- ✓ Mexican blend cheese (1 c.)
- ✓ Cilantro, chopped (.25 c.)

How to make:

1. Take out a small pan and get it prepared with a little butter.
2. When that is done, take out a bowl and mix in the cheese, salt, chilis, half and half and eggs. Pour this into a prepared pan and cover it up with some foil.
3. Pour a few cups of water into the inner part of your Instant Pot and add a trivet into it. Place your pan onto that trivet.
4. Lock the lid of the Instant Pot into place. Select the Manual function and adjust so the pressure is at High.
5. Cook this meal for about 20 minutes. When the cooking is done, give the cooker some time to release for a few minutes before finishing with the quick release method. Unlock the lid at this time.
6. Take the pan out of the Instant Pot and remove the foil. Scatter the rest of the cheese on top and place under a hot broiler for a few minutes.
7. Allow the frittata to sit for another ten minutes. Then use a knife to gently loosen the sides from the pan.
8. Place a plate on the pan and then invert the frittata onto the plate. Slice up before serving.

Nutritional information:

Calories: 283
Carbs; 7g
Protein: 16g
Fat: 22g

Egg Loaf

What's inside:

- ✓ Water (2 c.)
- ✓ Eggs (6)
- ✓ Butter

How to make:

1. Take out a heatproof bowl and use butter to grease it up really well.
2. Crack the eggs into this prepared bowl, trying to keep the yolks so they stay intact. Cover this bowl with some foil for now and set it to the side.
3. Pour some water into the inner cooking pot of your Instant Pot and then place a trivet on top. Place the foil-covered bowl of eggs onto this trivet as well.
4. Lock the Instant Pot lid in place. Select Manual and adjust so the pressure is on high.
5. Cook this for four minutes. Use the quick release method to get the air out of the pot.
6. Slowly take the bowl out of the pot and take the egg loaf out of it. Chop this up and use for a snack or meal or even in an egg salad.

Nutritional information

Calories: 74
Carbs: 0g
Protein: 6g
Fat: 5g

Cheesy Eggs

What's inside:

- ✓ Salt
- ✓ Mixed herbs (1 tsp.)
- ✓ Grated cheddar (2 Tbsp.)
- ✓ Milk (.25 c.)
- ✓ Eggs (3)

How to make:

1. Take out a heat proof bowl that will fit in your Instant Pot and cover it in nonstick spray.
2. Whisk together herbs, salt, milk, and eggs. Pour this into the bowl and then place that bowl into your steamer basket.
3. Add a cup of water to the bottom of the Instant Pot. Lower the basket into the Instant Pot.
4. Seal the pot and let it cook on a low pressure. After seven minutes, quickly let the steam out and take the lid off the pot.
5. Add the cheese and stir well. Let this rest for a bit and finish cooking all on its own.

Nutritional information:

Calories: 100
Carbs: 3g
Protein: 16g
Fat: 8g

Sausage Breakfast Casserole

What's inside:

- ✓ Soy sauce
- ✓ Mixed herbs (1 Tbsp.)
- ✓ Broth (1 c.)
- ✓ Onions and bell pepper mix, chopped (1 lb.)
- ✓ Chopped sausage, cooked (1 lb.)

How to make

1. Bring out the Instant Pot and place all of the ingredients inside, stirring to mix well.
2. Place the lid on top of the Instant Pot and press the Stew function to get started.
3. After ten minutes, the dish is done. Release the pressure naturally. Allow the dish to cool down before serving.

Nutritional information

Calories: 360
Carbs: 10g
Protein: 35g
Fat: 24g

Almond Flake Oats

What's inside:

- ✓ Nutmeg (1 Tbsp.)
- ✓ Cinnamon (1 Tbsp.)
- ✓ Powdered sweetener (2 Tbsp.)
- ✓ Milk (2 c.)
- ✓ Flaked almonds, mashed (.5 c.)

How to make:

1. Take out your Instant Pot and let it heat up. Pour the milk in the bottom to make a base.
2. When the milk warms up a bit, add in the rest of the ingredients, making sure to mix well.
3. Seal and close the vent on your lid and then choose the Manual setting to start cooking.
4. After five minutes, the dish is done. Allow the pressure to naturally release before serving.

Nutritional information

Calories: 380
Carbs: 11g
Protein: 15g
Fat: 18g

Sweet Chili Eggs

What's inside:

- ✓ Sugar free sweet chili sauce (2 Tbsp.)
- ✓ Cooked sausage (.25 c.)
- ✓ Milk (.25 c.)
- ✓ Eggs (3)

How to make:

1. Find a bowl that is heat resistant and will also fit into your Instant Pot. Spray it with some cooking spray.
2. In a different bowl, take some time to whisk together your sauce, milk, and eggs.
3. Pour this into your prepared bowl and add in the sausage. This bowl can then be placed in your steamer basket.
4. Add a cup of water to the bottom of the Instant Pot before lowering the basket inside.
5. Seal up the Instant Pot and cook this dish on a low pressure. After seven minutes, you can let the pressure out of the Instant Pot slowly.
6. Stir the dish one more time and allow it to finish cooking using its own heat before serving.

Nutritional information:

Calories: 165
Carbs: 6g
Protein: 19g
Fat: 11g

Eggs and Spinach

What's inside:

- ✓ Salt (1 pinch)
- ✓ Grated Parmesan (2 Tbsp.)
- ✓ Milk (.25 c.)
- ✓ Spinach (2 c.)
- ✓ Eggs (3)

How to make:

1. Take out a bowl that can stand the heat and will fit into the Instant Pot. Spray with some cooking spray.
2. In another bowl, you will need to whisk together the salt, milk, and eggs. Pour this egg mixture into your original bowl before placing that bowl into the steamer basket.
3. Add a cup of water to the base of your Instant Pot before lowering the basket into it as well.
4. Seal up the Instant Pot and cook the dish on a low pressure. After seven minutes, let the pressure come out naturally.
5. Once the pressure is gone, you can add in the Parmesan and spinach to the mixture.
6. Stir this together well and let the dish finish cooking with its own heat before you serve.

Nutritional information:

Calories: 110
Carbs: 4g
Protein: 16g
Fat: 8g

Tomato and Broccoli Delight

What's inside:

- ✓ Minced onion (1)
- ✓ Dry basil (1 Tbsp.)
- ✓ Broth (1 Tbsp.)
- ✓ Cherry tomato (1 lb.)
- ✓ Chopped broccoli (1 lb.)

How to make:

1. Take the broccoli, tomato, broth, dray basil, and minced onion and throw them into the Instant Pot.
2. Mix the ingredients together and then place the lid tightly on top, making sure it is secure.
3. Turn the Instant Pot onto the Stew setting and let it bake. After ten minutes, the dish is done.
4. Let the pressure release naturally from the Instant Pot before serving.

Nutritional information

Calories: 130
Carbs: 6g
Protein: 6g
Fat: 10g

Chicken and Egg Stew

What's inside:

- ✓ Mixed herbs (1 Tbsp.)
- ✓ Quartered hard boiled eggs (2)
- ✓ Broth (1 c.)
- ✓ Chopped vegetables (1 lb.)
- ✓ Shredded chicken, cooked (1 lb.)

How to make:

1. Bring out your Instant Pot and all the chicken, vegetables, broth, eggs, and herbs inside.
2. Stir these around before placing the lid on top and letting it cook at the Stew function.
3. After ten minutes, the dish will be done. You can turn off the Instant Pot and release the pressure naturally.

Nutritional information

Calories: 340
Carbs: 10g
Protein: 43g
Fat: 20g

Mushrooms and Pork

What's inside:

- ✓ Shredded cheddar (1 Tbsp.)
- ✓ Mixed herbs (1 Tbsp.)
- ✓ Mushroom soup (1 c.)
- ✓ Chopped mushrooms (1 lb.)
- ✓ Diced pork (1 lb.)

How to make:

1. Bring out your Instant Pot and add in the cheese, herbs, soup, mushrooms, and pork.
2. Stir these together and then place the lid on top to cook. Press the Stew button.
3. After 10 minutes, the dish is done and you can release the pressure naturally. Serve warm!

Nutritional information

Calories: 410
Carbs: 10g
Protein: 42g
Fat: 20g

Tomato and Chicken Stew

What's inside:

- ✓ Minced onion (1)
- ✓ Mixed herbs (1 Tbsp.)
- ✓ Chopped tomatoes (1 lb.)
- ✓ Vegetable broth (1 c.)
- ✓ Diced chicken, cooked (1 lb.)

How to make:

1. Take the onion, mixed herbs, vegetable broth, tomatoes, and cooked chicken and add them into the Instant Pot.
2. Mix the ingredients together well and then add the lid on top of the Instant Pot tightly.
3. Turn on the Instant Pot to the Stew function and let these ingredients cook together.
4. After 10 minutes, your dish is done and you can naturally release the pressure before serving.

Nutritional information:

Calories: 230
Carbs: 6g
Protein: 42g
Fat: 13g

Egg Fried Vegetables

What's inside:

- ✓ Herb and spice mix (2 Tbsp.)
- ✓ Milk (2 Tbsp.)
- ✓ Mixed vegetables (1 c.)
- ✓ Egg whites (4 oz.)

How to make:

1. Take out a bowl that is heat proof and will fit into your Instant Pot and spray it with some cooking spray.
2. In another bowl, whisk together your seasonings with the milk and eggs before pouring into the bowl and adding your vegetables.
3. Place this bowl into the steamer basket and pour a cup of water into the bottom of the Instant Pot as well.
4. Seal the Instant Pot and cook on a low pressure. After seven minutes have passed, you can depressurize this quickly.
5. Stir this well and then allow it to rest. This helps the meal to finish cooking using its own heat.

Nutritional information:

Calories: 100
Carbs: 7g
Protein: 15g
Fat: 1g

Ratatouille

What's inside:

- ✓ Vegetable stock (2 c.)
- ✓ Onion, chopped (1)
- ✓ Chopped zucchini (1)
- ✓ Beef tomatoes, chopped (2)
- ✓ Chopped eggplant (1)

How to make:

1. Bring out your Instant Pot and place the beef tomatoes, onion, zucchini, eggplant, and vegetable stock inside.
2. Stir the ingredients around and then place the lid on top as well. Turn this on to the Stew setting.
3. After ten minutes, you can let the pressure out quickly. Stir the ingredients around again before serving.

Nutritional information:

Calories: 100
Carbs: 7g
Protein: 3g
Fat: 2g

Herb Crusted Chicken

What's inside:

- ✓ Olive oil (2 Tbsp.)
- ✓ Chopped herps (.25 c.)
- ✓ Sugar snap peas (1 c.)
- ✓ Sweet pepper, chopped (1)
- ✓ Chopped chicken breast (2 oz.)

How to make:

1. Grab your chicken and pat it dry. Do the same with the vegetables. Place both of these into a bowl and then roll with a bit of oil.
2. After the chicken and vegetables are covered, add in the herbs and toss around as well.
3. Put the rest of the oil into your Instant Pot to heat up. Add in the vegetables and the chicken and cook.
4. After ten minutes, check to see if the chicken is cooked through. If it is, then serve warm.

Nutritional information:

Calories: 126
Carbs: 6g
Protein: 14g
Fat: 6g

Stuffed Mushrooms

What's inside:

- ✓ Pepper and salt
- ✓ Minced garlic clove (1)
- ✓ Minced onion (.5)
- ✓ Minced broccoli (.5 c.)
- ✓ Mushrooms without their stalks (10)

How to make:

1. Take your mushrooms and rinse them off.
2. Bring out a bowl and mix together the pepper, salt, garlic, onion, and broccoli. When this mixture is done, add it to the mushrooms, filling each up until the mixture is gone.
3. Add the mushrooms into the steamer basket of your Instant Pot. Add a cup of water into the bottom of the Instant Pot before inserting the steamer basket.
4. Push the Steam button and let these cook. After five minutes the mushrooms are done and you can let the pressure ego out quickly. Serve these right away.

Nutritional information:

Calories: 100
Carbs: 2g
Protein: 1g
Fat: 2g

Pulled Chicken

What's inside:

- ✓ BBQ sauce (1 c.)
- ✓ Broth 1 c.)
- ✓ Shredded onion (2)
- ✓ Chicken breast (1.5 lbs.)

How to make:

1. Take out the Instant Pot and get it all set up. When the Instant Pot is ready, you can add the BBQ sauce, broth, onions, and chicken into the pot to cook.
2. After these are ready, place the lid on top of the Instant Pot and seal it tight.
3. Press the Stew function on the Pot and let it cook. After 35 minutes, the dish is done and you can let the pressure release naturally.
4. When the pressure is gone, take the chicken out and shred it up. Serve right away.

Nutritional information:

Calories: 290
Carbs: 7g
Protein: 45g
Fat: 7g

Half Roast Chicken

What's inside:

- ✓ Broth (1 c.)
- ✓ Rub (2 Tbsp.)
- ✓ Mixed herbs (2 Tbsp.)
- ✓ Chicken (.5)

How to make:

1. Bring out a little bowl and mix together a bit of broth with the rub and the herbs.
2. Take this mixture and rub it all over the chicken until the chicken is covered completely.
3. Take out the Instant Pot and add the broth to the bottom. Then lower the chicken into the broth as well.
4. Place the lid on top of the Instant Pot and seal it up. Press the Stew button and let this cook.
5. After 35 minutes, the mixture should be done. Release the pressure naturally and then serve.

Nutritional information:

Calories: 300
Carbs: 6g
Protein: 43g
Fat: 9g

Turkey Meatball Stew

What's inside:

- ✓ Mixed seasoning (2 Tbsp.)
- ✓ Almond flour (3 Tbsp.)
- ✓ Chicken soup (1 c.)
- ✓ Chopped vegetables (1 lb.)
- ✓ Minced turkey (1 lb.)

How to make:

1. To start this recipe, bring out the Instant Pot and get it all set up.
2. Take the turkey and mix it together with the almond flour and the seasoning. Roll these into little balls.
3. Add the balls into the Instant Pot along with the vegetables and the chicken soup and add the lid on top.
4. Press the stew function and let this cook. After 35 minutes, naturally release the pressure before serving.

Nutritional information

Calories: 260
Carbs: 6g
Protein: 38g
Fat: 7g

Duck with Orange Sauce

What's inside:

- ✓ Marmalade (2 Tbsp.)
- ✓ Orange juice (1 c.)
- ✓ Broth (1 c.)
- ✓ Stir fry vegetables (1 lb.)
- ✓ Diced duck breast (1 lb.)

How to make:

1. Bring out the Instant Pot and give it time to heat up.
2. Add in the duck breast, vegetables, broth, orange juice, and marmalade to the Instant Pot and stir around.
3. Place the lid on top of your Instant Pot and then press the Stew button.
4. Allow this mixture to cook for 35 minutes. When that time is up, allow the pressure time to release naturally before serving.

Nutritional information:

Calories: 315
Carbs: 13g
Protein: 37g
Fat: 16g

Cilantro and Lemon Chicken

What's inside:

- ✓ Dry cilantro (2 Tbsp.)
- ✓ Juice from half a lemon
- ✓ Chicken broth (1 c.)
- ✓ Chopped vegetables (1 lb.)
- ✓ Chicken breast, diced (1 lb.)

How to make:

1. To start this recipe, dice up the chicken breast and chop the vegetables so they are ready to go.
2. Take out the Instant Pot and get it set up. When the Instant Pot is ready, add the cilantro, lemon juice, chicken broth, vegetables, and chicken breast inside.
3. Place the lid on top of the Instant Pot and make sure it is sealed. Cook on the Stew function.
4. After 35 minutes are done, let the pressure have time to release naturally and serve.

Nutritional information

Calories: 280
Carbs: 4g
Protein: 45g
Fat: 12g

Balsamic Turkey

What's inside:

- ✓ Balsamic reduction (2 Tbsp.)
- ✓ Chicken soup (1 c.)
- ✓ Chopped vegetables (1 lb.)
- ✓ Diced turkey breast (1 lb.)

How to make:

1. Bring out the Instant Pot and get it set up. Take some time to dice the turkey and chop up the vegetables as well.
2. When the Instant Pot is ready, add the turkey, vegetables, chicken soup and balsamic reduction inside.
3. Press the Stew function to begin cooking. After 35 minutes, you can let the pressure out naturally and then serve.

Nutritional information:

Calories: 295
Carbs: 5g
Protein: 46g
Fat: 14g

Salmon Bake

What's inside:

- ✓ Sea salt
- ✓ Juice from half a lemon
- ✓ Fish broth (1 c.)
- ✓ Mediterranean vegetables, chopped (1 lb.)
- ✓ Salmon (1 lb.)

How to make:

1. Take out a foil pouch and set it to the side. Add in the salmon, vegetables, lemon juice, and salt inside.)
2. Place this pouch into the steamer basket of the Instant Pot. Add the broth into the pot around the foil packet.
3. Place the lid on top of your Instant Pot and press the Steam function to get started.
4. After 15 minutes, let the pressure naturally release. Let this cool down before unwrapping the foil and enjoy.

Nutritional information:

Calories: 260
Carbs: 5g
Protein: 36g
Fat: 12g

Tuna Sweetcorn Casserole

What's inside:

- ✓ Spicy seasoning (2 Tbsp.)
- ✓ Vegetable broth (1 c.)
- ✓ Vegetables, chopped (1 lb.)
- ✓ Sweetcorn kernels (.5 lb.)
- ✓ Tuna (3 tins)

How to make

1. Prepare all of the ingredients. Get the Instant Pot out and make sure it is all set up.
2. Combine the spicy seasoning, vegetable broth, vegetables, sweetcorn, and tuna into the Instant Pot.
3. Place the lid on the Instant Pot, making sure that it is nice and tight. Push the Stew function to begin cooking.
4. After 35 minutes, this casserole is done. Allow the pressure to release naturally before serving.

Nutritional information

Calories: 300
Carbs: 6g
Protein: 43g
Fat: 9g

Shrimp Coconut Curry

What's inside:

- ✓ Ghee or oil (1 Tbsp.)
- ✓ Curry paste (3 Tbsp.)
- ✓ Coconut yogurt 1 c.)
- ✓ Sliced onion (1)
- ✓ Cooked shrimp (.5 lb.)

How to make:

1. Take out the Instant Pot and let it heat up a little bit. Once the Instant Pot is warmed up, add in the curry paste, oil, and onion to cook.
2. When you see that the onion is soft, you can add in the yogurt and shrimp to the pot as well.
3. Add the lid on top of the Instant Pot and seal it shut. Push the Stew function and let these cook.
4. After 20 minutes, the dish is done. You can release the pressure naturally before serving.

Nutritional information

Calories: 380
Carbs: 13g
Protein: 40g
Fat: 22g

Mussels and Spaghetti Squash

What's inside:

- ✓ Salt
- ✓ Crushed garlic (3 Tbsp.)
- ✓ Fish broth (1 c.)
- ✓ Spaghetti squash (.5)
- ✓ Shelled mussels, cooked (1 lb.)

How to make

1. Bring out a bowl and mix together the slat and garlic with the mussels until covered.
2. Place the prepared mussels inside the squash before adding both of them to the Instant Pot.
3. Pour the broth into the pot as well, making sure that it gets all around the other ingredients.
4. Place the lid on top of the Instant Pot and let it seal properly. Cook this on the stew function.
5. After 35 minutes, this dish is done. Give the pressure time to release naturally so it can cool down.
6. After the dish has had time to cool down, take the squash out and shred it up to make it into the spaghetti.
7. Serve these spaghetti noodles with the mussels and enjoy.

Nutritional information

Calories: 265
Carbs: 7g
Protein: 48g
Fat: 9g

Cod in White Sauce

What's inside:

- ✓ Black pepper (3 Tbsp.)
- ✓ Peas (1 c.)
- ✓ White sauce (2 c.)
- ✓ Swede and carrots, chopped (1 lb.)
- ✓ Cod fillets (1 lb.)

How to make:

1. Take some time to chop up all the vegetables and the cod fillets if you would like.
2. Once the Instant Pot is set up and ready to be used, add in the pepper, peas, white sauce, swede and carrots, and the cod fillets.
3. Add the lid on top of the Instant Pot and make sure that it is sealed properly.
4. Push the Stew function and let these ingredients cook together. After five minutes, it is time to release the pressure naturally. Serve this dish after the pressure is gone.

Nutritional information

Calories: 390
Carbs: 10g
Protein: 41g
Fat: 26g

Adobo Pork Chops

What's inside:

- ✓ Olive oil (3 Tbsp.)
- ✓ Minced garlic cloves (3)
- ✓ Squeezed lemon juice (.25 c.)
- ✓ Coconut aminos (.5 c.)
- ✓ Pork chops (1 lb.)

How to make:

1. Take all of your ingredients and add them into the Instant Pot. Season with some pepper and salt if you would like and then add .25 cups of water to the bottom.
2. Add the lid on top of the Instant Pot and get it all set up. Press the "Meat/Ste" button and let this cook.
3. After 50 minutes, do the natural pressure release option before serving this dish.

Nutritional information:

Calories: 271
Carbs: 2.3g
Protein: 18.2g
Fat: 23.3g

Mexican Pulled Pork

What's inside:

- ✓ Coconut oil (5 Tbsp.)
- ✓ Cumin powder (1 tsp.)
- ✓ Garlic powder (2 tsp.)
- ✓ Cinnamon (1 tsp.)
- ✓ Pork shoulder (4 lbs.)

How to make:

1. Take out the Instant pot and pour 1.5 cups of water inside the bottom. Add in the rest of the ingredients as well and season with some pepper and salt to taste.
2. Close the lid on the Instant Pot and then turn on the "Meat/Stew" function to heat it up.
3. This mixture needs about 90 minutes to cook. After this time, you can do the natural release pressure.
4. When the pressure is gone, open up the lid, take out the meat, and shred it up with a few forks before serving.

Nutritional information

Calories: 364
Carbs: 0.5g
Protein: 20.4g
Fat: 35.9g

Pork Vindaloo

What's inside:

- ✓ Lemon juice (3 Tbsp.)
- ✓ Water (1 c.)
- ✓ Garam masala (1 Tbsp.)
- ✓ Cubed pork shoulder (2 lbs.)
- ✓ Coconut oil (.25 c.)

How to make:

1. Turn on the Instant Pot and give it time to heat up. Add in the oil and the pork, letting it have time to sear on all sides for a few minutes.
2. After three minutes have passed, add in the garam masala. This can cook for a few minutes before you take the rest of the ingredients and mix them in as well.
3. Close the lid to the instead pot and press your Meat/Stew button to cook everything.
4. After 55 minutes, allow the pressure some time to release before serving.

Nutritional information:

Calories: 322
Carbs: 0.4g
Protein: 23.9g
Fat: 25.2g

Pork Coconut Curry

What's inside:

- ✓ Coconut milk (1 c.)
- ✓ Cubed pork shoulders (2 lbs.)
- ✓ Garam masala (1 Tbsp.)
- ✓ Minced garlic clove (3)
- ✓ Coconut oil (3 Tbsp.)

How to make:

1. Turn on the Instant Pot and let the oil heat up inside. Cook both the garam masala and the garlic until they become fragrant.
2. Add in the meat and give it time to sear on all sides, which will take about three minutes.
3. Add in the coconut milk before you close the lid to your Instant Pot and get it set up.
4. Press the Meat/Stew button and adjust your time. After 45 minutes, you can do the natural pressure release before serving.

Nutritional information

Calories; 371
Carbs: 1.8g
Protein: 23.4g
Fat: 28.7g

Pork Casserole

What's inside:

- ✓ Sliced mushrooms (1 c.)
- ✓ Water (1 c.)
- ✓ Yellow mustard (3 Tbsp.)
- ✓ Cubed pork shoulder (2 lbs.)
- ✓ Butter (4 Tbsp.)

How to make:

1. Turn on the Instant Pot and let it heat up. Add in the butter and give it time to melt.
2. When the butter is melting, add in the mustard and the pork shoulder. Cook and stir for the next three minutes.
3. Stir in the water and the mushrooms. Season with some pepper and salt before adding the lid on top.
4. Press the Meat/Stew button and let this mixture cook. After 50 minutes, you can use the natural pressure release and serve.

Nutritional information

Calories: 286
Carbs: 0.3g
Protein: 22.9g
Fat: 20.8g

Instant Pot Roast

What's inside:

- ✓ Pepper and salt
- ✓ Cayenne pepper flakes (1 Tbsp.)
- ✓ Liquid smoke (2 Tbsp.)
- ✓ Pork butt (4 lbs.)
- ✓ Olive oil (5 Tbsp.)

How to make

1. Take out your Instant Pot before adding in all of the ingredients along with a cup of water.
2. Put the lid on top of the Instant Pot and then seal it shut to help everything cook.
3. Press the Meat/Stew button and let this all cook for a bit.
4. After 90 minutes, the dish should be done. Do the natural pressure release and allow it to cool down before serving.

Nutritional information

Calories: 456
Carbs: 0.7g
Protein: 32.9g
Fat: 39g

Instant Pot Ribs

What's inside:

- ✓ Olive oil (5 Tbsp.)
- ✓ Smoked paprika (1 Tbsp.)
- ✓ Onion powder (1 Tbsp.)
- ✓ Garlic powder (1 Tbsp.)
- ✓ Baby back ribs (1 rack)

How to make:

1. Add the baby back ribs onto a baking sheet. Season them with the rest of your ingredients, and then add on a bit of pepper and salt to taste at the end.
2. Rub the ribs so they are coated on all sides with this spice mixture before placing them in the Instant Pot.
3. Pour in half a cup of water before putting the lid on top and getting everything sealed up.
4. Press the Slow Cook button on your Instant Pot and let this cook for a bit. After eight hours, the meal is done and you can serve.

Nutritional information

Calories: 700
Carbs: 3.2g
Protein: 49g
Fat: 50g

Pork Chops

What's inside:

- ✓ Chicken broth (.5 c.)
- ✓ Heavy cream (.5 c.)
- ✓ Pork chops (6)
- ✓ Minced garlic cloves (3)
- ✓ Butter (8 Tbsp.)

How to make:

1. Turn on the Instant Pot so it has time to heat up a bit. Add in the garlic and the butter and cook for a few minutes.
2. When those are done, add in the pork chops. These need to be seared for three minutes on each side.
3. Add in the broth and the heavy cream to the mixture and season with the pepper and salt.
4. Close the lid on your Instant Pot and then seal the lid well. Press the Meat/Stew button.
5. After 30 minutes, you can quickly release the pressure and then serve warm.

Nutritional information:

Calories: 439
Carbs: 0.9g
Protein: 26.7g
Fat: 46.2g

Shredded Beef

What's inside:

- ✓ Pepper and salt
- ✓ Pasta sauce (2 c.)
- ✓ Bay leaves (2)
- ✓ Olive oil (2 Tbsp.)
- ✓ Diced stewing beef (3 lbs.)

How to make:

1. Take out the Instant Pot and set it on a high setting. Add in a bit of oil.
2. Season your beef with some pepper and salt and then brown the meat on all sides.
3. When the meat is browned, cover it with the sauce and the bay leaves. Then seal the lid on tight.
4. Select a Manual setting and let this cook for a bit. After 60 minutes, slowly let the pressure out of the Instant Pot.
5. Let the beef have some time to set before you remove and shred the beef. Serve warm.

Nutritional Information

Calories: 318
Carbs: 2g
Protein: 21g
Fat: 16g

Tasty BBQ Loaf

What's inside:

- ✓ Vegetable broth (1 c.)
- ✓ Crushed cornflakes (1 c.)
- ✓ Eggs (2)
- ✓ BBQ sauce (.5 c.)
- ✓ Lean ground beef (3 lbs.)

How to make:

1. Take out a bowl and mix together the meat, eggs, and crumbs until well combined.
2. Take out your Instant Pot and add the steam rack inside. Pour in the broth.
3. Form the mixture in the bowl into a loaf and cover it up with the BBQ sauce. Wrap it all up in some aluminum foil.
4. Place this prepared meatloaf onto a steam rack and place the lid of the Instant Pot on tight.
5. Steam this for the next 30 minutes. When that time is done, release the pressure and give the meatloaf some time to cool down before removing and serving.

Nutritional information

Calories: 488
Carbs: 11g
Protein: 25g
Fat: 27g

Simple Chili

What's inside:

- ✓ Oil (2 Tbsp.)
- ✓ Beef broth (1 c.)
- ✓ Chopped tomatoes (28 oz.)
- ✓ Mixed beans (1.5 c.)
- ✓ Ground beef (1.5 lbs.)

How to make:

1. Take out the Instant Pot and turn it onto a high setting. Add the oil and give it some time to heat up.
2. When the oil is warm, add the beef and give it time to brown all the way through.
3. Add in the rest of your ingredients, making sure to mix well.
4. When those ingredients are warm, seal up the Instant Pot and let it cook on the Stew setting.
5. After 25 minutes have passed, the meal should be done. Release the pressure and let it rest for 5 minutes before removing.

Nutritional information

Calories: 188
Carbs: 4g
Protein: 11g
Fat: 10g

Thai Ribs

What's inside:

- ✓ Coconut oil (3 tsp.)
- ✓ Diced onion (1)
- ✓ Curry powder (2 Tbsp.)
- ✓ Pureed tomatoes (4)
- ✓ Beef ribs (3 lbs.)

How to make:

1. Take the curry powder and rub it all over your ribs. Place them into a little baggie and set them in the fridge so they have time to marinate through the night.
2. When you are ready to make, get the Instant Pot out and set it on medium. Add in some oil and the onion and cook for a few minutes.
3. Add in the ribs, going in small batches, until they are browned, and then set aside.
4. Mix together the remainder of your ingredients in the Instant Pot to make them warm.
5. When the sauce is hot, add the ribs to the Pot and put the lid on tight. Cook on the Meat setting.
6. After 20 minutes, the meat is done. Release the pressure naturally and give the meat about five minutes to rest before removing. Serve these warm.

Nutritional information:

Calories: 410
Carbs: 14g
Protein: 22g
Fat: 18g

Country Beef

What's inside:

- ✓ Beef broth (1 c.)
- ✓ Dry red wine (1 c.)
- ✓ Sliced mushrooms (.5 c.)
- ✓ Sliced carrots (2)
- ✓ Cubed round steak (5 lbs.)

How to make:

1. Take out the Instant Pot and set it on a high setting. Heat up a tablespoon of oil.
2. When the oil is warm, add in the beef and let it brown on all sides.
3. When the beef is browned, you can stir in the rest of the ingredients, stirring to deglaze.
4. Place the lid on the Instant Pot and cook on the Stew setting. When 20 minutes are up, slowly release the pressure.
5. Allow the dish to rest for about 5 minutes before removing and serving warm.

Nutritional information

Calories: 384
Carbs: 6g
Protein: 24g
Fat: 32g

Spicy Turkey Tacos

What's inside:

- ✓ Worcestershire sauce (1 Tbsp.)
- ✓ Beef broth (1.25 c.)
- ✓ Mexican seasoning (4 Tbsp.)
- ✓ Olive oil (1 Tbsp.)
- ✓ Ground turkey meat (1 lb.)

How to make:

1. Take out the Instant Pot and set it to a high level. Heat up the olive oil inside.
2. When the oil is nice and warm, add in the ground turkey and let it become browned on all sides.
3. Add in the rest of the ingredients before placing the lid on top. Set this to the Stew setting.
4. After five minutes, you can let the pressure out from the Instant Pot quickly and give it a few minutes to cool down.
5. Serve with some lettuce taco shells and any toppings you would like.

Nutritional information:

Calories: 233
Carbs: 2g
Protein: 11g
Fat: 13g

Orange Balsamic Chicken

What's inside:

- ✓ Balsamic vinegar (2 Tbsp.)
- ✓ Orange juice (1 c.)
- ✓ Chicken breasts 6)
- ✓ Minced garlic (.5 tsp.)
- ✓ Thyme (.5 tsp.)

How to make:

1. Take out a bowl and combine the garlic and the thyme. Use a pestle and mortar to help crush these two ingredients together.
2. Rub this mixture on all parts of the chicken before placing into your Instant Pot.
3. Mix the vinegar and orange juice and pour it on top of the chicken. Place the lid on the Instant Pot nice and tight.
4. Using your Slow Cook function, cook this meal. After three hours, naturally release the pressure.
5. Let it set for a few minutes before serving and enjoy!

Nutritional information

Calories: 383
Carbs: 12g
Protein: 14g
Fat: 18g

Easy Tamari Chicken

What's inside:

- ✓ Edamame (.66 c.)
- ✓ Rinsed long grain rice (1 c.)
- ✓ Mixed vegetables (2 c.)
- ✓ Tamari (.66 c.
- ✓ Chicken breasts (2)

How to make:

1. Take out your Instant Pot and get it all set up. Place the rice into a bamboo nest in the steamer basket for your pot.
2. Take the rest of the ingredients and mix them in the Instant Pot before placing the lid on top.
3. Seal the lid and pick the Stew setting. After 16 minutes, the dish is done and you can do a natural release of the pressure.
4. Allow the dish to have about five minutes to rest before you serve.

Nutritional information:

Calories: 287
Carbs: 5g
Protein: 11g
Fat: 13g

Hot and Spicy Chicken

What's inside:

- ✓ Black beans (.5 c.)
- ✓ Buffalo wings hot sauce (3 c.)
- ✓ Sweet corn (.5 c.)
- ✓ Sliced pineapple (.5 c.)
- ✓ Chicken breasts (2 lbs.)

How to make:

1. Take your chicken and slice it up into some nice strips. Add these to a bowl with the rest of the ingredients, making sure everything is coated well.
2. Take out the Instant Pot and set it on a high setting. When the Instant Pot is hot, add in the chicken.
3. Seal the lid and set to the Meat setting. Cook this for about 30 minutes.
4. After this time, quickly release the pressure and allow the meal some time to cool down before serving.

Nutritional Information

Calories: 418
Carbs: 15g
Protein: 16g
Fat: 22g

Lamb for Dinner

What's inside:

- ✓ Mint sauce (.5 c.)
- ✓ Broth (1 c.)
- ✓ Carrots, chopped (2)
- ✓ Onion, quartered (1)
- ✓ Lean lamb, diced (1 lb.)

How to make:

1. Take out the Instant Pot and get it set up. Place the lamb on the bottom of the pot.
2. Place the carrots and the onion all around your lamb and then pour your sauce and broth on top of everything.
3. Place the lid on top of the Instant Pot and then push the Stew setting.
4. After 35 minutes, the meal will be done. Slowly release the pressure naturally and then serve!

Nutritional Information

Calories: 400
Carbs: 14g
Protein: 37g
Fat: 20g

Shredded Beef

What's inside:

- ✓ Mixed spices (2 Tbsp.)
- ✓ Gravy (1 c.)
- ✓ Lean steak (1.5 lbs.)

How to make:

1. Take out the Instant Pot and mix together all of your ingredients. Stir them around well.
2. Place the lid on top of the Instant Pot nice and tight. Press the Stew function to begin cooking.
3. After 35 minutes, the meal is finished. Use the slow release method to get the pressure out.
4. Take the steak out of the pressure cooker and shred it up before serving.

Nutritional information:

Calories: 200
Carbs: 2g
Protein: 48g
Fat: 5g

Italian Sausage Casserole

What's inside:

- ✓ Mixed herbs (1 Tbsp.)
- ✓ Broth (1 c.)
- ✓ Mediterranean vegetables (1 lb.)
- ✓ Cooked sausages, chopped (1 lb.)

How to make:

1. Take out the Instant Pot and get everything set up. Take some time to chop up the vegetables and sausages.
2. Add all the ingredients into the Instant Pot and stir to combine well.
3. Place the lid on top of the Instant Pot and press the Stew function to get the cooking started.
4. After five minutes, you can let the pressure release naturally and then serve the meal.

Nutritional information:

Calories: 320
Carbs: 8g
Protein: 41g
Fat: 18g

Roast Beef

What's inside:

- ✓ Gravy (1 c.)
- ✓ Beef broth (1 c.)
- ✓ Winter vegetables, cubed (1 lb.)
- ✓ Beef joint, trimmed (1 lb.)

How to make:

1. Take out a small bowl and mix together the gravy and the broth. Add the beef into the bottom of the Instant Pot.
2. Pour your gravy and broth mixture on top of the beef and then add the vegetables into the pot as well.
3. Place the lid on top of your Instant Pot and then press the Stew function to begin cooking.
4. After an hour, let the pressure release naturally and then serve.

Nutritional information:

Calories: 275
Carbs: 5g
Protein: 49g
Fat: 7g

Beef Stew

What's inside:

- ✓ Black pepper
- ✓ Beef broth (1 c.)
- ✓ Chopped vegetables (1 lb.)
- ✓ Diced stewing steak (1 lb.)

How to make:

1. Bring out your Instant Pot and get everything set up. Add the pepper, broth, vegetables, and steak inside.
2. Stir these ingredients around and then add the lid to the Instant Pot. Press the Stew function.
3. After 35 minutes, the stew should be done. Let the pressure release naturally and then serve.

Nutritional information

Calories: 300
Carbs; 6g
Protein: 43g
Fat: 9g

Mashed Cauliflower

What's inside:

- ✓ Salt and pepper
- ✓ Juice from half a lemon
- ✓ Olive oil (2 Tbsp.)
- ✓ Butter (.5 c.)
- ✓ Chopped cauliflower (1 head)

How to make:

1. Take out your Instant Pot and add a steam rack to it. Place a cup of water in the bottom of the pot.
2. Add your cauliflower florets into the steak rack and close the lid, making sure it is on tight.
3. Press your Steam function and let these cook for a bit.
4. After seven minutes, the cauliflower is done and you can use the quick pressure release.
5. After the cauliflower has some time to cool down, you can place it in the food processor along with the remainder of the ingredients.
6. Pulse these ingredients together until they are nice and smooth before serving.

Nutritional information

Calories: 41
Carbs: 2.4g
Protein: 0.7g
Fat: 4.9g

Cauliflower Fried Rice

What's inside:

- ✓ Coconut aminos (5 Tbsp.)
- ✓ Beaten egg (1)
- ✓ Chopped onions (2)
- ✓ Sesame oil (2 Tbsp.)
- ✓ Halved cauliflower (1 head)

How to make:

1. Take out your Instant Pot and place a steam rack into the bottom of it. Add in a cup of water as well.
2. When that is ready, add in the cauliflower florets to your steam rack and place the lid tightly on top.
3. Press your Steam button and adjust the time to go for seven minutes. When this time is up, do a quick release of the pressure.
4. Take the cauliflower out and then clean up the Instant Pot to have it ready for later.
5. Place your cauliflower into a food processor and pulse until it becomes grainy in texture.
6. Turn the Instant Pot back on and heat up the oil. Stir in the onions until they are fragrant.
7. Now add in the eggs, breaking them up into small pieces, along with the coconut aminos and the cauliflower rice.
8. Adjust the seasonings as you would like them to be and then serve this dish warm.

Nutritional information

Calories: 108
Carbs: 4.3g
Protein: 3.4g
Fat: 8.2g

Avocado Devilled Eggs

What's inside:

- ✓ Cilantro, chopped (3 Tbsp.)
- ✓ Smoked paprika (.25 tsp.)
- ✓ Garlic powder (.25 tsp.)
- ✓ Avocado, pitted and the meat scooped out (1)
- ✓ Eggs (6)

How to make:

1. Take out your Instant Pot and add in 1.5 cups of water along with the eggs. Put the lid on top, making sure that it is nice and tight.
2. Press the Manual function and let these cook. After six minutes, the eggs will be done and you can do a quick pressure release.
3. Give the eggs time to cool down completely before you crack them and peel off the shells.
4. Slice your eggs going lengthwise and scoop out the yolk. Place this yolk in a mixing bowl and add the paprika, garlic powder, and avocado.
5. Season this mixture with some pepper and salt if you would like and mix until it is well combined.
6. Fill the hollows of your egg whites with this avocado mixture, garnish with cilantro, and serve.

Nutritional information

Calories: 184
Carbs: 4.1g
Protein: 9.6g
Fat: 14.5g

Spinach Quiche Bites

What's inside:

- ✓ Pepper and salt
- ✓ Beaten eggs (8)
- ✓ Chopped spinach (2 c.)
- ✓ Chopped onion (1)
- ✓ Coconut oil (2 Tbsp.)

How to make:

1. Take out the Instant Pot and let it heat up a bit. Add on the oil and the onion and cook a few minutes.
2. Stir in the spinach now and let it wilt for a minute. When the spinach is wilting a bit, pour in the eggs and season with some pepper and salt.
3. Close the lid and make sure that it is on nice and tight. Press your Slow Cook button and adjust the time.
4. After 4 hours, allow the pressure to release and the quiche to cool down.
5. When you are ready to serve these, slice them up into smaller bites and enjoy!

Nutritional information

Calories: 112
Carbs: 2.1g
Protein: 6.3g
Fat: 9.7g

Chinese Eggplant

What's inside:

- ✓ Coconut oil (4 Tbsp.)
- ✓ Minced garlic (3 cloves)
- ✓ Grated ginger (1 tsp.)
- ✓ Coconut aminos (.25 c.)
- ✓ Sliced eggplants (2)

How to make:

1. Take out the Instant Pot and get it all set up. Add in all the ingredients and season with some pepper and salt. You can add some more water if it's needed.
2. After stirring a bit, close the lid and make sure it is on tight. Press your Slow Cook button.
3. After 5 hours, the dish is done and you can serve.

Nutritional information

Calories: 385
Carbs: 35g
Protein: 5.8g
Fat: 28.3g

Garlic Wings

What's inside:

- ✓ Pepper (1 tsp.)
- ✓ Salt (1 tsp.)
- ✓ Garlic powder (1 Tbsp.)
- ✓ Avocado oil (2 Tbsp.)
- ✓ Chicken wings (12)

How to make:

1. Take out your Instant Pot and get it all set up. Place all of your ingredients inside.
2. After stirring these a bit, close the lid and make sure it is on tight. Press the Slow Cook button.
3. This dish will need to cook for 6 hours before serving.

Nutritional information

Calories: 61
Carbs: 1g
Protein: 6.6g
Fat: 13.2g

Chicken Tortilla Soup

What's inside:

- ✓ Heavy whipping cream (1 c.)
- ✓ Chicken broth base, powdered (1 Tbsp.)
- ✓ Poultry seasoning (1 tsp.)
- ✓ Mixed frozen vegetables (1 bag)
- ✓ Diced chicken thighs (1 lb.)

How to make:

1. Take out your Instant Pot and add in some salt and pepper with the chicken broth base, poultry seasoning, two cups of water, vegetables, and chicken.
2. Lock the lid in place and select the Manual setting. Make sure the pressure is on high and cook these ingredients together for 2 minutes.
3. When the cooking is done, use the quick release method to help get it cooled off.
4. Unlock the lid and then stir in the cream. Serve warm when ready.

Nutritional information

Calories: 327
Carbs: 13g
Protein: 26g
Fat: 19g

Cinnamon Butter Bites

What's inside:

- ✓ Beaten eggs (5)
- ✓ Almond flour (1 c.)
- ✓ Cinnamon (1 Tbsp.)
- ✓ Liquid stevia (.25 c.)
- ✓ Unsalted butter (1 stick)

How to make:

1. Mix all of your ingredients together in a bowl and season them with some salt.
2. Take out the Instant Pot and then grease one of the inner pots as well. Pour in the batter.
3. Place the lid on top of the Instant Pot and then press your Slow Cook button to start.
4. After five hours, this dish is done. Allow the pressure to come out and serve warm.

Nutritional information:

Calories: 161
Carbs: 1.2g
Protein: 4.5g
Fat: 15.5g

Almond Bread

What's inside:

- ✓ Baking powder (1.5 tsp.)
- ✓ Erythritol (1.5 c.)
- ✓ Almond flour (2.5 c.)
- ✓ Olive oil (.25 c.)
- ✓ Beaten eggs (3)

How to make:

1. Take out a bowl and mix together all of the ingredients. Add in a bit of cinnamon or salt if you would like.
2. Once you have time to mix the batter properly, grease up the Instant Pot and pour the batter inside.
3. Close the lid on the pot and make sure it is on nice and tight. Press the Slow Cook button to start.
4. After five hours, you can use the quick release method to get rid of all the steam. Take the bread out and give it time to cool down before serving!

Nutritional information

Calories: 67
Carbs: 0.6g
Protein: 1g
Fat: 7g

Chocolate Pudding

What's inside:

- ✓ Salt
- ✓ Liquid stevia (.5 tsp.)
- ✓ Cacao powder (2 Tbsp.)
- ✓ Chia seeds (.25 c.)
- ✓ Coconut milk (1 c.)

How to make:

1. Take all of your ingredients and pour them into the prepared Instant Pot. Stir them all around well.
2. Add the lid on top of the Instant Pot and get it all set up before pressing the Slow Cook button.
3. Let this dish cook on that setting for three hours before serving.

Nutritional information

Calories: 346
Carbs: 21.2g
Protein: 8.4g
Fat: 27.5g

Coconut Boosters

What's inside:

- ✓ Coconut flakes, dried (.25 c.)
- ✓ Erythritol (1 tsp.)
- ✓ Vanilla (1 tsp.)
- ✓ Chia seeds (.5 c.)
- ✓ Coconut oil (1 c.)

How to make:

1. Bring out your Instant Pot and let it get heated up. Once it is warm, you can add in the coconut flakes, erythritol, vanilla, chia seeds, and the coconut oil.
2. Stir these ingredients around for a bit. After five minutes, you can scoop these into balls and place onto a baking sheet.
3. After the mixture is all scooped up, place into the fridge to set for a few hours before serving.

Nutritional information

Calories: 480
Carbs: 9.4g
Protein: 2.9g
Fat: 50g

Keto Brownies

What's inside:

- ✓ Erythritol (2 tsp.)
- ✓ Almond flour (.25 c.)
- ✓ Dark chocolate chips (.33 c.)
- ✓ Beaten eggs (5)
- ✓ Coconut oil (.5 c.)

How to make

1. For this recipe, bring out a mixing bowl and combine all the ingredients together, adding in a bit of salt if you would like.
2. Pour this mixture into a prepare Instant Pot and then put the lid on top, ensuring that the lid is on tight.
3. Press the Slow Cook button and let the mixture cook. It needs to go for 5 hours on this setting.
4. When the time is up, release the pressure from the pot and give the brownies some time to cool before serving.

Nutritional information

Calories: 214
Carbs: 3.4g
Protein: 5.4g
Fat: 20.7g

Vanilla Jell-O

What's inside:

- ✓ Vanilla (1 tsp.)
- ✓ Heavy cream (1 c.)
- ✓ Erythritol (3 Tbsp.)
- ✓ Gelatin powder (2 Tbsp.)
- ✓ Boiling water (1 c.)

How to make:

1. Take out your Instant Pot and place some boiling water inside. Press so the pot is on and let the water get up to a simmer.
2. Add the gelatin at this time and give it some room to dissolve. Once the gelatin is dissolved, stir in the remainder of the ingredients.
3. At this time, pour the mixture into some Jell-O molds and put into the fridge to set for a few hours before enjoying.

Nutritional information

Calories: 105
Carbs: 5.2g
Protein: 3.3g
Fat: 7.9g

Keto Fudge

What's inside:

- ✓ Erythritol (4 Tbsp.)
- ✓ Baking powder (.5 tsp.)
- ✓ Cocoa powder (.25 c.)
- ✓ Melted butter (1 stick)
- ✓ Beaten eggs (6)

How to make

1. To start this recipe, bring out a bowl and add all the ingredients inside. Add in a bit of salt as well.
2. Mix these ingredients together well and then pour them into a prepared Instant Pot.
3. Add the lid to the top and make sure it is on tight. Press the Slow Cook button and let the fudge cook.
4. After four hours, you can do a quick release of the pressure and allow the fudge some time to cool down before serving.

Nutritional information

Calories: 131
Carbs: 1.3g
Protein: 4.3g
Fat: 12.2g

Peanut Butter Cookies

What's inside:

- ✓ Baking soda (1 pinch)
- ✓ Applesauce (1 Tbsp.)
- ✓ Powdered sweetener (2 Tbsp.)
- ✓ Chocolate chips (.33 c.)
- ✓ Peanut butter (.33 c.)

How to make:

1. Take out a bowl and mix together the baking soda, applesauce, and sweetener.
2. After these are combined, add in the peanut butter and then fold in the chocolate chips.
3. Find a tray that is heat proof and is going to fit into the steamer tray of your Instant Pot.
4. Make your cookies and place them on this heat proof tray.
5. Pour a cup of water into the bottom of the Instant Pot. And then lay the tray into the steamer basket. Lower the steamer basket into the bottom of your Instant Pot.
6. Place the lid on top of the Instant Pot and make sure it is on time. Turn the pot onto the steam function.
7. After 20 minutes, the cookies will be done. Let the pressure out quickly and when the cookies have time to cool, serve.

Nutritional information

Calories: 390
Carbs: 20g
Protein: 10g
Fat: 26g

Keto Custard

What's inside:

- ✓ Water (1 c.)
- ✓ Caramel sauce (1.5 tsp.)
- ✓ Powdered sweetener (1.5 Tbsp.)
- ✓ Cream cheese (2 oz.)
- ✓ Eggs (2)

How to make:

1. Take out a blender and place the eggs, cream cheese, water, caramel sauce, and powdered sweetener and blend everything together well.
2. Pour this into a heat proof bowl that is going to fit well inside your Instant Pot.
3. Pour a cup of water into the Instant Pot and place the bowl into the steamer basket inside the pot.
4. Add the lid on top and use your Steam function for this one. Cook for the next 20 minutes.
5. After this time, let the pressure out quickly before serving.

Nutritional information

Calories: 273
Carbs: 1.5g
Protein: 9g
Fat: 27g

White Chocolate

What's inside:

- ✓ Hot water
- ✓ White chocolate mix (3 tsp.)
- ✓ Powdered sweetener (6 tsp.)
- ✓ Double cream (4 Tbsp.)

How to make:

1. Set up the Instant Pot before mixing together the hot water, double cream, sweetener, and white chocolate mix inside.
2. Place the lid on top of the Instant Pot and press the Stew function.
3. After two minutes have passed, use the natural release method to let all of the steam and pressure out of the pot.
4. After this has had time to cool down, stir the mixture well and serve.

Nutritional information

Calories: 105
Carbs: 3g
Protein: 4g
Fat: 12g

Cooking Notes

CPSIA information can be obtained
at www.ICGtesting.com
Printed in the USA
LVHW050755180319
611005LV00006B/353/P